I0505789

Nephrology Study Guide

Concise Information That Every Med Student, Physician, NP, and PA Should Know

Just the facts are included in this book. This is the perfect text if you are looking for a quick review of the information you need to know about Nephrology. This rapid access information won't waste your time. This Nephrology Study Guide has distilled the key details down to the concise facts that you will understand and remember.

This Nephrology Study Guide is an ideal resource for medical students and anyone who wants to understand more about internal medicine. This book quickly reviews the information about the most common Nephrology questions and answers.

Did you know the pathophysiology of contrast induced renal failure?

Did you know that renal artery stenosis accounts for approximately of 4% of cases of hypertension?

Did you know that RBC casts reflect glomerular inflammation or ischemia?

The Nephrology Study Guide will present this information and the other key details about Nephrology in a way that you will find useful for patient care, clinical rotations, and board review.

Buy this book now if you want this quick and concise information about Nephrology.

Copyright © 2013; Chart-MD - All rights reserved.

This Kindle book contains material protected under International and Federal Copyright laws and Treaties. Any unauthorized reprint or use of this material is prohibited. Unauthorized duplication or distribution of this material in any form is strictly prohibited. Violators will be prosecuted to the fullest extent of the law. No part of this publication may be reproduced, stored in a retrieval system or transmitted in any form or by any means, electronic, mechanical, photocopying, recording or otherwise, without prior written permission from the author/publisher. The author, publisher, and distributor of this product assume no responsibility for the use or misuse of this product, or for any physical or mental injury, damage and/or financial loss sustained to persons or property as a result of using this system. The liability, negligence, use, misuse or abuse of the operation of any methods, strategies, instructions or ideas contained in the material herein is the sole responsibility of the reader.

Disclaimer

All the material contained in this book is provided for educational and informational purposes only. No responsibility can be taken for any results or outcomes resulting from the use of this material.
While every attempt has been made to provide information that is both accurate and effective, the author does not assume any responsibility for the accuracy or use/misuse of this information.

Acknowledgements

I dedicate this book to my beautiful wife and children, who I love more than all the water in all the oceans and all the seas.

Chapter 1: Questions and Answers

What is reflected by WBC casts in the urine?

WBC casts in the urine reflect inflammation in the renal interstitium (i.e. pyelonephritis) RBC casts reflect glomerular inflammation or ischemia

What is an autosomal dominant disease characterized by bilateral enlargement of kidneys secondary to multiple large cysts. Patients present with hematuria, pain, hypertension, and progressive renal failure. What is this disease?

Adult polycystic kidney disease

Which autosomal recessive disease is characterized by bilateral enlargement of kidneys with presence of multiple small cysts within the collecting ducts at right angle to the cortex? It is associated with multiple liver cysts.

Childhood polycystic kidney disease (autosomal recessive)

What three conditions are associated with adult polycystic kidney disease?

Polycystic liver disease

Berry aneurysms

Mitral valve prolapse

What are the three steps to treating myoglobinuria?

Volume repletion with IVF Mannitol diuresis

Alkalinize urine with IV bicarbonate

What are three potential symptoms of hypokalemia?

Weakness Tetany Ileus

What is the break down the body fluid composition by location?

Fluids = 60% of Total body composition; 40% = intracellular fluid; 20% = extracellular fluid (15% interstitial, 5% plasma)

What are five treatments of hyperkalemia?

Ca gluconate (cardio protective)

Na bicarbonate (alkalosis drives K into cells) Glucose + insulin

Kayexalate and Lasix

Dialysis

List three signs on physical exam of hyperkalemia?

Decreased DTR's

Weakness

Respiratory failure

What is the etiology of stenosis in renal artery stenosis?

2/3 secondary to atherosclerosis

1/3 secondary to fibromuscular dysplasia

What are 4 signs of hyponatremia?

Seizure

Coma

Nausea and vomiting

Ileus

What are four symptoms of hypernatremia?

Seizures

Confusion

Pulmonary or peripheral edema

Respiratory paralysis

What are three signs of hypermagnesemia?

Respiratory failure CNS depression Diminished DTR's

How can you think of renal tubular acidosis with respect to potassium levels?

Type I has a low serum potassium

Type II has normal serum potassium

Type IV has high serum potassium

Which two drugs interfere with the test for creatinine and can result a falsely increased creatinine?

Cefoxitin

Acetone

List 3 drugs known to increase the creatinine by interfering with the secretion of creatinine?

Cimetidine

Trimethoprim

Probenecid

What are the common EKG changes seen in hypomagnesemia?

Prolonged PR or QT intervals, T-wave flattening or inversion ST straightening

What are the two types of lactic acidosis?

Type A lactic acidosis is secondary to hypoxemia or hypo perfusion. Type B is secondary to systemic illness (sepsis, liver disease, and diabetes), ingestion of drugs, or congenital errors of metabolism.

What are four causes of post-renal renal failure?

Urethral obstruction Ureteral obstruction Bladder outlet obstruction

What are four causes of glomerulonephritis?

Post streptococcal

IgA nephropathy

Rapidly progressive glomerulonephritis

Crescentic glomerulonephritis

What are four etiologies of nephrotic syndrome?

Minimal change disease

Focal segmental glomerulosclerosis

Membrane glomerulonephropathy

Membranoproliferative glomerulonephritis

What is the four general mechanisms of hyperkalemia?

Increased dietary intake

Decreased excretion

Cell lysis

Transmembrane cellular shifts

What are the two general mechanisms of hypernatremia?

Hypernatremia with hypovolemia (disorders of thirst, renal loss, extra-renal loss)

Hypernatremia with normal or expanded volume

Hypernatremia in the hospitalized patient is generally iatrogenic

What are the two mechanisms of metabolic acidosis?

Hydrogen ions added to the serum

Loss of bicarbonate

What are four common mechanisms of pre-renal renal failure?

Intravascular volume depletion

Renal vasoconstriction

Peripheral vasodilatation

Cardiac disease

Describe four findings of HIV nephropathy?

Increased frequency in African Americans

Heavy proteinuria

Large echogenic kidneys

Rapidly progresses to end stage renal disease

Besides renal associated findings, what are 4 other organ systems associated with autosomal dominant polycystic kidney disease?

Liver cysts and other abdominal organ cysts

Berry aneurysms at the Circle of Willis

Mitral valve prolapse

Diverticulosis and diverticulitis

Which analgesics are associated with analgesic nephropathy?

Phenacetin and acetaminophen are associated

Aspirin is not associated

What are four common findings a presentation of RPGN?

Oliguria Hypertension Edema

Active sediment with erythrocytes and casts

What are the common findings of IgA nephropathy?

Asymptomatic microscopic hematuria/proteinuria

Gross hematuria post exercise or viral illness

What are the common findings at presentation of acute glomerulonephritis?

Decreased GFR Oliguria Hypertension

Active urine sediment

Proteinuria which is rarely nephrotic range

What are three risk factors for renal vein thrombosis?

Nephrotic syndrome

Tumors invading the renal veins

Hypercoagulable state

What are four common findings at presentation of membranous nephropathy?

Edema

Hypertension

Microalbuminemia

Normal GFR

What are the four common findings at presentation of focal segmental glomerulosclerosis?

Nephrotic syndrome (66%)

Hypertension

Microscopic hematuria

Decreased GFR (30-40%)

What are the four findings of nephrotic syndrome?

Urine protein of greater than 3-3.5 g/dl

Hypoalbuminemia

Edema

Hyperlipidemia

What are the 4 mechanisms of proteinuria?

Overflow of elevated normal or abnormal serum proteins

Decreased reabsorption of normal filtered proteins Increased glomerular permeability

Changes in renal hemodynamics

What are the ECG findings in Hyperkalemia?

Tenting of T-waves in II, III, V2, V3, V4

Widening of QRS S-T depression

Flattening of P-wave PR prolongation

Eventual degeneration into V-Fib

What are the ECG findings of hypercalcemia?

Shortened QT interval (normal is 0.12-0.20 seconds) Absence of ST segment

Early peak of T waves

Gradually descending T waves

To delay onset of ESRD in patients with diabetic nephropathy, what are four clinical tactics?

Decrease BP to below 130/85 (will decrease proteinuria, prevent progression from microalbuminemia to overt nephropathy)

Use ACE inhibitors

Dietary protein restriction to 0.6-0.8 g/kg

Maintain strict glycemic control

Describe the renal physiology of creatinine?

Primarily filtered in the glomerulus

Also with significant tubular secretion

Remember that creatinine clearance overestimates the GFR

List the four main etiologies of end stage renal disease?

DM (33%) --5 year survival is less than 20% Essential HTN (30%)

Glomerulonephritis (15%) Polycystic kidney disease (5%)

What are the electrolyte concentrations in normal saline?

154 Na

154 Cl

What are three of the body's responses to hypovolemia?

Sodium retention via rennin--angiotensin

Water retention via ADH

Vasoconstriction via angiotensin II and sympathetics

What are 5 indications for dialysis in the setting of renal failure?

Fluid overload

Refractory hyperkalemia

BUN > 130

Acidosis

Pericardial friction rub

What percentage of the population will develop nephrolithiasis?

1-5%

Is nephrolithiasis more common in men?

Yes, more common 2:1

Which RPGN is characterized by antiglomerular basement membrane antibodies?

Type I RPGN

Which RPGN is characterized by immune complex deposits?

Type II RPGN

Which RPGN is commonly called pauci immune and is not characterized by immune complexes or anti-GBM Antibodies?

Type III RPGN

Which type of RPGN is characterized by antibodies directed against the alpha-3 chain of type IV collagen with linear deposits of immunoglobulin along the glomerular basement membrane? This RPGN is also associated with Goodpasture's syndrome?

Type I RPGN

Which type of rapidly progressive glomerular nephritis (RPGN) is commonly associated with a positive ANCA?

Type III (paucimmune)

What are common findings associated with analgesic nephropathy?

Nocturia, polyuria, sterile pyuria, predisposition to volume depletion, renal colic, hematuria, and hypertension

Describe the laboratory evaluation of urine of patients with hepatorenal syndrome

The FENA will be <1%, the Urine sodium will be < 10 mEq/L, and the urinary sediment will be normal

What are two signs of hypocalcemia?

Chvostek's sign---facial muscle spasm with tapping of facial nerve

Trousseau's sign---carpal spasm after occluding flow to the forearm with the blood pressure cuff

What are four EKG changes found in hypokalemia?

Premature atrial contractions

Premature ventricular contractions

T-wave flattening

Presence of U-waves

What are four EKG changes in hyperkalemia?

Peaked T waves

Prolonged P-R

Wide QRS with bradycardia

V-fib with asystole

What are the signs and symptoms of hypercalcemia?

Stones

Bones

Abdominal groans

Psychiatric overtones

What are the most common causes of hypercalcemia?

Hypercalcemia can be caused by calcium supplements, hyperparathyroidism, immobility, iatrogenic, metastasis, milk alkali syndrome, Paget's disease, Addison's, acromegaly, cancer, Zollinger Ellison. excessive vitamin D, excessive vitamin A, and sarcoid.

What is one common finding among all three renal tubular acidosis?

They are all associated with a normal gap acidosis

Which type of renal tubular acidosis is associated with multiple myeloma?

Multiple myeloma is associated with a type 2 RTA

Which type of RTA is associated with diabetic nephropathy?

Diabetes is associated with a type IV RTA

In the setting of hypoalbuminemia for which you are correcting the serum calcium, what correction to you need to make for the ionized calcium?

The ionized calcium is not altered by the serum albumin, therefore no correction is needed for a low albumin.

What is the most important clue to the diagnosis of methanol toxicity?

Disturbed vision (formic acid inhibits cytochrome oxidase in optic nerves, reducing flow of axoplasm resulting in ischemic nerve damage)

A serum osmolality > 10 indicates one of two things?

Decreased serum water per volume of sample being measured (hyperlipidemia, hyperproteinemia)

Increased serum concentration of low molecular weight particles such as mannitol, methanol, ethylene glycol, ETOH, or paraldehyde

What are the typical laboratory findings in methanol toxicity?

Anion gap acidosis Na - (Cl + HCO3)

Osmolar gap greater than 10 (Osm gap = measured - calculated) Measured - (2 x Na) + BUN/2.8 + Glu/18

What is the characteristic complement levels in patients with renal disease with cryoglobulinemia and hepatitis C?

Hypocomplementemia C1q-C4

What is the formula for calculating serum osmolality?

2 x Na + BUN/2.8 + Glucose/18

In IgA nephropathy, these patients commonly present with hematuria a few days after URI or GI infection. What are the complement levels?

Normal C4 and C3 levels

Which electrolyte imbalance is likely to occur in patients with metabolic acidosis?

Hyperkalemia

What is the most common renal complication of autosomal dominant polycystic kidney disease?

Hypertension

Name one drug commonly associated with distal renal tubule acidosis?

Amphotericin B is known to cause a type I RTA

How do you measure the anion gap?

NA - (Cl + HCO3)

How do you measure the fractional excretion of sodium (FENA)?

Urine sodium x Serum creatinine/ Serum sodium x Urine creatinine x 100

<1 is prerenal

What is the specific target of the anti-GBM antibodies in Goodpasture's syndrome?

The alpha-3 chain of type IV collagen

How can the administration of bicarbonate cause worsening of hypocalcemia?

NaHCO3 can decrease ionized calcium by increasing calcium binding to albumin

What illness commonly presents with arthralgia, purpura, abdominal pain, microscopic hematuria, mild proteinuria, azotemia, and proliferative glomerulonephritis characterized by IgA deposits?

Henoch-Schonlein purpura

What is the mechanism of renal artery stenosis as a cause of hypertension?

Stenosis of renal artery results in decreased perfusion of the JG apparatus and activation of the aldosterone-renin-angiotensin system (Etiology of 4% of HTN)

Which disease can be characterized by headache, diastolic HTN, flank bruits (50%), and decreased renal function?

Renal artery stenosis

What are the findings in a patient with hypomagnesemia?

Vomiting, anorexia, paresthesia, muscle cramps, confusion

Milk alkali syndrome is caused by ingestion of excessive amounts of absorbable antacids (> or = to 5 grams of calcium daily) and is characterized by three findings?

Hypercalcemia

Alkalosis

Renal insufficiency

Explain the effect of magnesium deficiency on other electrolytes?

Magnesium deficiency impairs calcium and potassium metabolism

Magnesium is coenzyme in ATP (Na/K pump) and deficiency results in intracellular K deficiency

What are the 4 effects of hyperkalemia on the EKG?

Tent shaped T-waves Decreased or absent p waves Short QT interval

Widening QRS complex

What is the effect of hypocalcemia on the ECG?

QT interval prolongation

Flat or inverted T-waves

What is the effect of hypercalcemia on the heart?

Short or absent ST segment

Decreased QT interval

What are the mechanisms of hypocalcemia?

Renal insufficiency, hypoalbuminemia, vitamin D deficiency, hypomagnesemia, pancreatitis, hyperphosphatemia, osteoblastic metastasis, idiopathic hyperparathyroidism, sepsis

Describe 3 important findings in post streptococcal glomerulonephritis following pharyngitis?

6-20 day latent period

ASO >250 u/ml

Low C3

What are 4 findings in Hepatorenal syndrome?

Azotemia

Hyponatremia

Progressive oliguria

Hypotension

What are the three reasons for hypercoaguable state in nephrotic syndrome (particularly membranous glomerulonephritis)?

AT-III and alpha 2 antitrypsin are lost in the urine

Factor VIII, Von Willibrand factor, Fibrinogen, Factor V, and Factor VII accumulate in the blood plasma

Abnormalities in platelet function

What are the findings of methanol ingestion?

Systemic acidosis

Direct neurotoxicity (secondary to the metabolites formic acid and formaldehyde)

What is the most common intrinsic renal disease that leads to acute renal failure?

Acute tubular necrosis

What is the most common cause of acute renal failure in hospitalized patients?

Pre-renal azotemia

What is the most common cause of death in patients with acute tubular necrosis?

Hyperkalemia

What is the most common cause of hypocalcemia in the setting of acute renal failure?

Hyperphosphatemia

What is the BUN to Creatinine ratio in patients with dehydration?

Approximately 15-20 to 1

What is the BUN to Creatinine ratio in patients with post-renal renal failure?

Approximately >10 to 1

What is the BUN to Creatinine ratio in patients with intrinsic renal failure?

The BUN and Creatinine rise proportionally in these patients resulting in approximately a 10/1 ratio

What is the daily production of creatinine by the body?

The body produces approximately 15-30 mg/kg/day of creatinine

How quickly will the creatinine rise in the setting of complete renal failure?

The creatinine will rise approximately 1-2 mg/dL per day

What should be suspected if the rate of increase of creatinine is greater than 3 mg/dL per day?

The patient should be evaluated for another source of creatinine such as muscle

Can cephalosporins affect the serum creatinine measurement?

Cephalosporins can result in a false increase in the serum creatinine through interference with the Jaffe reaction used in the labs for measurement of creatinine

Can dobutamine affect the serum creatinine measurement?

Dobutamine can falsely decrease the serum creatinine

Can diabetic ketoacidosis affect the serum creatinine measurement?

Diabetic ketoacidosis can interfere with the testing for serum creatinine resulting in a false elevation

What are three factors in limiting progression of chronic renal failure in Type I diabetics with chronic renal failure?

ACE inhibitors

Dietary protein restriction

Careful control of serum glucose levels

What is the normal 24-hour urine protein secretion?

< 150 mg/day

Describe the definition of microalbuminuria?

Excretion of 30-300 mg/dl of albumin

What is the definition of hematuria?

Greater than 3-5 red cells per high power field

What percent of adult idiopathic nephrotic syndrome is caused by minimal change disease?

20%

What is the most common etiology of nephrotic syndrome in African Americans?

Focal segmental glomerulosclerosis

What are the most common etiologies of focal segmental glomerulosclerosis?

Idiopathic, heroin. HIV, infection, sickle cell, obesity, and urine reflux

What is the most common etiology of nephrotic syndrome among Caucasians?

Membranous nephropathy

What are six common etiologies of membranous nephropathies?

Idiopathic, syphilis, Hepatitis B, SLE, gold salts, and malignancy

What is the most common etiology of nephrotic syndrome associated with thrombosis?

Membranous nephropathy

What is the most common form of idiopathic glomerulonephritis?

IgA nephropathy

What is the most common cause of hypocalcemia?

Chronic renal failure

Hyperglycemia is the most common cause of hyperosmolar hyponatremia. How do you correct the serum sodium for hyperglycemia?

Each 100 mg/dl of increased glucose causes a 1.6 mEq/liter decrease in serum sodium. Treatment is directed at correcting the serum glucose.

What percentage of adults by the age of 50 y/o will develop simple or solitary renal cysts?

25-30%

What are 6 common findings in autosomal dominant polycystic kidney disease?

Flank or back pain, gross hematuria, abdominal mass, frequent UTI's, hypertension, and nephrolithiasis

What percentage of patients with polycystic kidney disease develop adenocarcinoma of the kidney?

1.50%

What are 5 common findings in patients with medullary sponge kidney?

Common findings include microscopic/gross hematuria, hypercalciuria, nephrocalcinosis, and calcium stones. This disease is not associated with decreased GFR

What is the most common etiology of end stage renal disease in the United States?

Diabetes mellitus

What is the term used to describe nodular intercapillary glomerulosclerosis in patients with diabetes?

Kimmelsteil-Wilson nodules

What is the pathogenesis of aminoglycoside induced renal failure?

These antibiotics disrupt the membrane phospholipids in tubular cells leading to cell damage

What is the pathophysiology of contrast induced renal failure?

Radiocontrast agents induce intrarenal vascular constriction resulting in ischemia to epithelial cells

What is the most common underlying renal pathology of nephrotic syndrome in patients with solid tumors?

Membranous glomerulopathy

Which common cause of adult end stage renal disease is inherited autosomal dominant and is related to a mutation on the short arm of chromosome 16?

Polycystic kidney disease

Hyperkalemia can be due to decreased GFR only if GFR is below what level?

GFR < 20 ml/min

What is the primary cause of volume overload in end stage renal disease?

Volume overload occurs because of inability of kidney to excrete sodium. It usually only occurs with oliguric acute renal failure and ESRD

Describe the mechanisms of hyperkalemia in renal failure?

GFR < 20ml/min, Type IV RTA, Ace inhibitors, NSAIDS, Salt substitute, Fruit frenzy, Oral penicillin

What is the probable diagnosis in a patient with hyponatremia, urine osmolarity > serum osmolarity, with a urinary sodium> 30 meq/l, and a normal BUN/Creatinine?

SIADH

What are the 24 hour sodium and potassium requirements?

Sodium: 1.0 meq/kg/24 hours

Potassium: 1.5 meq/kg/day

What is the water requirements for 24 hours?

30-35 ml/kg/24 hours

What is the normal daily water losses in urine?

1.2-1.5 liters

What is the normal daily water losses in sweat?

200-400 ml

What are the normal daily water losses in feces?

100-200ml

What percentage of kidney stones are radio opaque?

90%

What is the most likely diagnosis in a patient with positive Chvostek's and/or Trousseau's sign and leg cramps?

Hypocalcemia

What is the most common organism causing acute bacterial pyelonephritis?

E. coli

What is the effect of a low magnesium on serum potassium and calcium?

Hypomagnesemia can result in hypocalcemia and hypokalemia

Describe the FENA in the setting of glomerulonephritis?

The FENA will be <1

What percentage of patients with polycystic kidney disease will develop cerebral aneurysms?

1-5%

How can a urine osmolality differentiate between SIADH and psychogenic polydipsia?

In SIADH the urine is concentrated and in psychogenic polydipsia the urine will be dilute

In the setting of hyponatremia, what happens if the serum sodium is corrected too quickly?

The intracellular sodium will not keep pace with the rising extracellular sodium, resulting in cell shrinkage and a neurologic disorder called central pontine myelinolysis

Is there a type III RTA?

No

This renal tubular acidosis (RTA) decreases bicarbonate reabsorption in the proximal tubule?

Type II RTA

Which RTA effects the Na/K/H exchange in the distal tubule, resulting in a hyperkalemic, hyperchloremic, normal gap acidosis?

Type 4 RTA

Which RTA is associated with a distal defect in the hydrogen ion secretion, resulting in hypokalemia, and normal gap acidosis?

Type I RTA

What is the most common type of kidney stone?

2/3 are calcium stones (calcium oxalate, calcium phosphate)

Which type of kidney stone is associated with urinary tract infections, particularly with urease producing bacteria such as Proteus, Pseudomonas, and Staphylococcus?

Struvite stones (staghorn calculi)

Describe the laboratory evaluation of complement in IgG and IgM mediated glomerulonephritis?

There will be low levels of C3 and C4

How does hypercalcemia cause polyuria and polydipsia?

This occurs secondary to calcium effect on the Na-K-Cl cotransport in the kidney which is similar to the furosemide effect at the same cotransport

Why is cortisol deficiency associated with hyponatremia?

Cortisol negatively modulates the release of ADH, so a deficiency in cortisol can lead to SIADH, and hyponatremia

Describe the osmolar gap in patient with metabolic acidosis secondary to methanol ingestion?

In the setting of methanol ingestion, there will be an increased osmolar gap (measured serum osmolarity - calculated serum osmolarity)

What are 6 intra-renal causes of acute renal failure?

The 6 most common intra-renal causes of acute renal failure are microvascular disease, macro vascular disease, intrarenal tubular obstruction, ATN, acute interstitial nephritis, or glomerulonephritis.

What is the pathogenesis and management of hyponatremia secondary to fulminant hepatic failure?

Hepatic failure leads to impaired free water clearance. This is managed by close monitoring of blood electrolyte and fluid balance along with free water restriction.

Why is it important to determine the serum osmolality in patients presenting with hyponatremia?

Sodium is the major extracellular cation. A patient presenting with hyponatremia should be hypoosmolar. If the patient is not hypoosmolar then other low molecular weight particles such as methanol, ethylene glycol, alcohol, or paraldehyde are present.

What is central pontine myelolinolysis?

A demyelinating process identified in the pons associated with hyponatremia. This occurs when hyponatremia is corrected too rapidly. Patients with chronic hyponatremia should not be corrected by no more than 12 meq in the first 24 hours.

What are the risk factors for poor neurological outcome in patients with hyponatremia?

The risk factors for poor neurological outcome include diuretic-induced hyponatremia, malnutrition, liver disease, hypoxia, alcoholism, and female gender

Although serum magnesium does not always correlate with intracellular magnesium levels, at what serum magnesium do people generally become symptomatic from hypomagnesemia?

Patients usually are not symptomatic unless serum magnesium falls below 0.5 mmol/L (1.2 mg/dL).

What is the effect of hypomagnesemia on calcium and potassium metabolism?

Magnesium deficiency impairs calcium and potassium metabolism. It is coenzyme in ATP (Na/K pump) and deficiency results in intracellular K deficiency.

What is the result of rapid correction of hyperglycemia with insulin in diabetics on the serum magnesium?

The insulin results in the magnesium entering the cell with the glucose hypomagnesemia commonly occurs.

Is there a clue to glucose control in a diabetic in the serum magnesium level?

The serum magnesium generally falls when glycosuria is present and the degree of hypomagnesemia can be a indication of poor glucose control

What is pseudohyperkalemia?

This occurs when there is falsely elevated potassium secondary to blood drawing techniques. Hemolysis resulting from trauma, fist clenching, and tissue damage can occur. Other etiologies include extreme leukocytosis or thrombocytosis.

How do you correct calcium for hypoalbuminemia?

For each 1 gram decrease in albumin you correct the calcium by increasing by 0.8 mg/dL.

What is the usual effect of malignancy related hypercalcemia on the endogenous PTH levels?

Malignancy related hypercalcemia will decrease endogenously released PTH.

What is the mechanism of hypercalcemia and sarcoidosis?

Elevated levels of 1, 25-dihydroxyvitamin D (calcitriol) produced by macrophages in the granulomas leads to increased calcium absorption in the intestine resulting in hypercalciuria and at times hypercalcemia

What is calciphylaxis?

Seen in end stage renal disease, secondary hyperparathyroidism, and high calcium phosphate product. It is characterized by vascular calcification in the tunica media of blood vessels resulting in painful violaceous skin lesions and ischemic necrosis

What is the most sensitive test for acute tubular necrosis?

The fractional excretion of sodium (FENA)

What conditions result in a FENA of <1%?

Perennial azotemia, acute glomerulonephritis, hepatorenal syndrome, and renal transplant rejection are associated with a FENA of less than 1%

What conditions result in a FENA of >1%?

Acute tubular necrosis, chronic uremia, and diuretics are associated with a FENA >1%

How often will patients with nonoliguric ischemic or nephrotoxic acute renal failure have a FENA of <1%?

Approximately 15% of patients will have this

Describe how to differentiate between hemoglobinuria and myoglobinuria?

Myoglobin (smaller than hemoglobin) is filtered by the kidneys, so urine will be discolored by the myoglobin but the serum will not. Hemoglobin is not as filtered, so the serum will be abnormal in appearance and the urine will be normal in appearance

What is the most common type of glomerulonephritis worldwide?

IgA nephropathy

What is the definition of oliguria and anuria?

Oliguria is <400 ml of urine per 24 hours and anuria is less than 100 ml urine per 24 hours

What underlying diagnosis is suggested in a patient with acute renal failure and white blood cells or white blood cell casts?

Interstitial nephritis

What underlying diagnosis is suggested in a patient with acute renal failure and red blood cell casts in the urine?

Glomerulonephritis

What is the definition of chronic renal failure?

Chronic renal failure is defined as renal function between 5-25% of normal

What is the definition of end stage renal disease?

End stage renal disease is present when the patient has less than 5% of normal renal function

What amount of proteinuria per day is indicative of nephrotic syndrome?

Proteinuria of more than 3.5 grams/day is indicative of nephrotic syndrome

What is the most common cause of hematuria of glomerular origin?

IgA nephropathy

What is the most common cause of type IV renal tubular acidosis (RTA?)

Hyporeninemic hypoaldosteronism

What is a common cause of metabolic alkalosis?

Volume contraction from diuretics or vomiting

When metabolic alkalosis occurs because of volume contraction, how does the serum chloride typically respond?

The urinary chloride is typically low (<10 meq/L) because the kidney is holding onto NaCl because the body is volume depleted

Which type of renal tubular acidosis is associated with nephrolithiasis and hypercalciuria?

Type I RTA

Which type of renal tubular acidosis is associated with multiple myeloma?

Type II RTA

Which type of renal tubular acidosis is associated with diabetic nephropathy?

Type IV RTA

What is the most common cause of hypokalemia?

Diuretics

How do you correct the serum calcium level for a low albumin?

For each decrease in albumin of 1, you should increase the serum calcium by 0.7 to obtain the corrected calcium

Is the ionized calcium affected by changes in the serum albumin?

No

Is there a difference in the effects of furosemide and thiazide diuretics on the calcium excretion by the kidney?

Yes, furosemide increase calcium excretion by the kidney and thiazide diuretics decrease calcium excretion by the kidney

Can diarrhea result in a metabolic acidosis?

Yes, diarrhea can cause a metabolic acidosis with an increased Chloride level. This is because bicarbonate is lost in the stool

Can thiazide diuretics result in a metabolic alkalosis?

Yes, thiazide diuretics can result in a metabolic alkalosis with a high urinary chloride level

What is the effect of lithium on the kidney?

Lithium can result in a nephrogenic diabetes insipidus by interfering with the kidney's ability to concentrate urine

What is stage I hypertension?

Stage I hypertension is characterized by a SBP of 140-159 or a DBP of 90-99 averaged from 2 or more readings on two or more occasions

What is stage II hypertension?

Stage II hypertension is SBP of 160-179 or DBP of 100-109 averaged from 2 or more readings from 2 or more occasions

What is stage III hypertension?

SBP greater than 180 or DBP >110 averaged from 2 or more readings from 2 or more occasions

What types of renal failure are characterized by a fractional excretion of sodium (FENA) of <1?

Pre-renal azotemia and acute glomerulonephritis can both have a low FENA. Acute glomerulonephritis will have an active urine sediment

What type of renal failure can be caused by volume depletion, atheroemboli, ACE inhibitors, and NSAIDs?

Pre-renal renal failure is associated with all of these conditions

In patients with pre-renal azotemia, would you expect the urine osmolality to be high or low?

Pre-renal azotemia is associated with a high urine osmolality

In patients with pre-renal azotemia, would you expect the urine sodium to be increased or decreased?

The urine sodium in pre-renal azotemia is generally decreased <20

What type of renal failure can be caused by acute tubular necrosis, rhabdomyolysis, lymphoma, methotrexate, cisplatin, aminoglycosides, and contrast dye?

Intra-renal renal failure

Would you expect the FENA to be elevated or low in patients with intra-renal renal failure?

These patients generally have a FENA <1

Would you expect the urine sodium to be elevated or low in patients with intra-renal renal failure?

These patients generally have an elevated urinary sodium >20

What is the most common cause of intra-renal renal failure?

Acute tubular necrosis

What is the most common cause of intra-renal renal failure?

Acute tubular necrosis

What are the most common causes of acute tubular necrosis?

ATN is most commonly cause by ischemia or toxic injury

What type of RTA can be associated with amphotericin B?

Type I RTA

What are the classic urinary findings of acute tubular necrosis?

Muddy brown granular casts

Which chemotherapy is associated with hemolytic uremic syndrome?

Mitomycin C

What is the BUN to Creatinine ratio in patients with dehydration?

Approximately 15-20 to 1

What is the BUN to Creatinine ratio in patients with post-renal renal failure?

Approximately >10 to 1

What is the BUN to Creatinine ratio in patients with intrinsic renal failure?

The BUN and Creatinine rise proportionally in these patients resulting in approximately a 10/1 ratio

What is the daily production of creatinine by the body?

The body produces approximately 15-30 mg/kg/day of creatinine

How quickly will the creatinine rise in the setting of complete renal failure?

The creatinine will rise approximately 1-2 mg/dL per day

What should be suspected if the rate of increase of creatinine is greater than 3 mg/dL per day?

The patient should be evaluated for another source of creatinine such as muscle

Can cephalosporins affect the serum creatinine measurement?

Cephalosporins can result in a false increase in the serum creatinine through interference with the Jaffe reaction used in the labs for measurement of creatinine

Can diabetic ketoacidosis affect the serum creatinine measurement?

Diabetic ketoacidosis can interfere with the testing for serum creatinine resulting in a false elevation

What is the most sensitive test for acute tubular necrosis?

The fractional excretion of sodium (FENA)

What conditions result in a FENA of <1%?

Prerenal azotemia, acute glomerulonephritis, hepatorenal syndrome, and renal transplant rejection are associated with a FENA of less than 1%

What conditions result in a FENA of >1%?

Acute tubular necrosis, chronic uremia, and diuretics are associated with a FENA >1%

How often will patients with nonoliguric ischemic or nephrotoxic acute renal failure have a FENA of <1%?

Approximately 15% of patients will have FENA < 1%

What are common findings associated with analgesic nephropathy?

Nocturia, polyuria, sterile pyuria, predisposition to volume depletion, renal colic, hematuria, and hypertension

Chapter 2: Fast Facts

Fact: Childhood polycystic kidney disease is an autosomal recessive disease characterized by bilateral enlargement of kidneys with presence of multiple small cysts within the collecting ducts at right angle to the cortex.

Fact: Adult polycystic kidney disease is an autosomal dominant disease characterized by bilateral enlargement of kidneys secondary to multiple large cysts. Patients present with hematuria, pain, hypertension, and progressive renal failure.

Fact: Cephalosporins can result in a false increase in the serum creatinine through interference with the Jaffe reaction used in the labs for measurement of creatinine.

Fact: Prerenal azotemia, acute glomerulonephritis, hepatorenal syndrome, and renal transplant rejection are associated with a
FENA of less than 1%.

Fact: EKG Changes of hypokalemia: Premature atrial contractions; premature ventricular contractions; T-wave flattening; Presence of U-waves.

Fact: Prerenal azotemia, acute glomerulonephritis, hepatorenal syndrome, and renal transplant rejection are associated with a FENA of less than 1%.

Fact: Nephrotic syndrome is characterized by proteinuria associated with hypoalbuminemia, hyperlipidemia, and edema.

Fact: In the setting of methanol ingestion, there will be an increased osmolar gap (measured serum osmolarity - calculated serum osmolarity).

Fact: Analgesic nephropathy is commonly associated with nocturia, polyuria, sterile pyuria, predisposition to volume depletion, renal colic, hematuria, and hypertension.

Fact: Type III (paucimmune) is commonly associated with a positive ANCA.

Fact: Type I RPGN is characterized by antibodies directed against the alpha-3 chain of type IV collagen with linear deposits of immunoglobulin along the glomerular basement membrane. This RPGN is also associated with Goodpasture's syndrome.

Fact: Type III RPGN is commonly called pauci immune and is not characterized by immune complexes or anti-GBM antibodies. Fact: Type II RPGN is characterized by immune complex deposits.

Fact: Hypocalcemia can develop because of renal insufficiency, hypoalbuminemia, vitamin D deficiency, hypomagnesemia, pancreatitis, hyperphosphatemia, osteoblastic metastasis, idiopathic hyperparathyroidism, or sepsis. Fact: Nephrolithiasis is more common in men 2:1.

Fact: The 6 most common intra-renal causes of acute renal failure are microvascular disease, macrovascular disease, intrarenal tubular obstruction, ATN, acute interstitial nephritis, and glomerulonephrotic disease.

Fact: Polyuria in patients with hypercalcemia is secondary to calcium effect on the Na-K-Cl cotransport in the kidney.
Fact: Renal artery stenosis accounts for approximately of 4% of cases of hypertension.

Fact: If serum osmolality is corrected too rapidly in patients with hyponatremia, intracellular sodium will not keep pace with the rising extracellular sodium, resulting in cell shrinkage and a neurologic disorder called central pontine myelinolysis.

Fact: Common findings of medullary sponge kidney include microscopic/gross hematuria, hypercalciuria, nephrocalcinosis, and calcium stones. This disease is not associated with decreased GFR.

Fact: Magnesium deficiency impairs calcium and potassium metabolism. Since magnesium is coenzyme in ATP (Na/K pump), deficiency of magnesium results in intracellular K deficiency.

Fact: Calciphylaxis is seen in end stage renal disease, secondary hyperparathyroidism, and a high calcium phosphate product. It is characterized by vascular calcification in the tunica media of blood vessels resulting in painful violacious skin lesions.

Fact: Nocturia, polyuria, sterile pyuria, predisposition to volume depletion, renal colic, hematuria, and hypertension are common findings associated with analgesic nephropathy.

Fact: Methanol toxicity is associated with: -Anion gap acidosis with an osmolar gap greater than 10.

Fact: Disturbed vision is a clue to methanol toxicity (formic acid inhibits cytochrome oxidase in optic nerves, reducing flow of axoplasm resulting in ischemic nerve damage).

Fact: Myoglobin (smaller than hemoglobin) is filtered by the kidneys, so urine will be discolored by the myoglobin but the serum will not. Hemoglobin is not as easily filtered, so the serum will be abnormal in appearance and the urine will be normal in appearance.

Fact: Hypercalcemia can develop in patients with sarcoidosis because elevated levels of 1, 25-dihydroxyvitamin D (calcitriol) produced by macrophages in the granulomas leads to increased calcium absorption in the intestine.

Fact: Hypocalcemia is associated with Chvostek's sign characterized by facial muscle spasm with tapping of facial nerve. Fact: Trousseau's sign is characterized by carpal spasm after occluding flow to the forearm with the blood pressure cuff.

Fact: The serum magnesium generally falls when glycosuria is present. The degree of hypomagnesemia can be an indication of poor glucose control.

Fact: Each 100 mg/dl of increased glucose causes a 1.6 mEq/liter decrease in serum sodium. Treatment of hyponatremia in the setting of hyperosmolar hyperglycemia is directed at correcting the serum glucose.

Fact: Magnesium decency impairs calcium and potassium metabolism. Magnesium is a coenzyme in ATP (Na/K pump) and deficiency results in intracellular K deficiency.

Fact: The risk factors for poor neurological outcome in patients with hyponatremia include diuretic-induced hyponatremia, malnutrition, liver disease, hypoxia, alcoholism, and female gender.

Fact: Central pontine myelolinolysis is a demyelinating process identified in the pons associated with hyponatremia. CPM occurs when hyponatremia is corrected too rapidly. Patients with chronic hyponatremia should not be corrected by no more than 12 meq.

Fact: Sodium is the major extracellular cation. A patient presenting with hyponatremia should be hypoosmolar. If the patient is not hypoosmolar then other low molecular weight particles such as methanol, ethylene glycol, alcohol, or paraldehyde are present.

Fact: The common EKG changes seen in hypomagnesemia include prolonged PR or QT intervals and T-wave flattening or inversion, and ST straightening.

Fact: Hypercalcemia can be caused by calcium supplements, hyperparathyroidism, immobility, iatrogenic, metastasis, milk alkali syndrome, Paget's disease, Addison's, acromegaly, cancer, Zollinger Ellison, excessive vit D, excessive vit A, and sarcoidosis.

Fact: An osmolar gap indicates the presence of accumulated osmolytes such as alcohol, radiocontrast, acetone, ethylene glycol, or methanol.

Fact: Hepatic failure leads to impaired free water clearance and hyponatremia. This is managed by close monitoring of blood electrolyte and fluid balance along with free water restriction.

Fact: Pseudohyperkalemia occurs when there is falsely elevated potassium secondary to blood drawing techniques. Fact: Hemolysis resulting from trauma, fist clenching, and tissue damage can occur.

Fact: Urine protein of greater than 3-3.5 g/dl, hypoalbuminemia, edema, and hyperlipidemia are the four findings of nephrotic syndrome.

Fact: Volume overload occurs in end stage renal disease because of inability of kidney to excrete sodium. It usually only occurs with oliguric acute renal failure and ESRD.

Fact: Edema, hypertension, microalbuminemia and a normal GFR are common findings at presentation of membranous nephropathy.

Fact: The common findings of IgA nephropathy are asymptomatic microscopic hematuria/proteinuria and gross hematuria post exercise or viral illness.

Fact: Oligouria, hypertension, edema, and active sediment with erythrocytes and casts are common findings a presentation of
RPGN.

Fact: WBC casts in the urine reflect inflammation in the renal interstitium (ie. Pyelonephritis). RBC casts reflect glomerular inflammation or ischemia.

Fact: Nephrotic syndrome (66%), hypertension, microscopic hematuria, and decreased GFR (30-40%) are common findings at presentation of focal segmental glomerulosclerosis.

Fact: Hydrogen ions added to the serum and loss of bicarbonate are the two mechanisms of metabolic acidosis. Fact: Urethral obstruction, ureteral obstruction, and bladder outlet obstruction are causes of post-renal renal failure.

Fact: Type A lactic acidosis is secondary to hypoxemia or hypoperfusion. Type B is secondary to systemic illness (sepsis, liver disease, and diabetes), ingestion of drugs, or congenital errors of metabolism.

Fact: Phenacetin and acetaminophen are associated with analgesic nephropathy. Aspirin is not associated.

Fact: Stage I hypertension is characterized by a SBP of 140-159 or a DBP of 90-99 averaged from 2 or more readings at two or more times.

Fact: 154 Na and 154 Cl are the electrolyte concentrations in normal saline.

Fact: Three risk factors for renal vein thrombosis are nephrotic syndrome, tumors invading the renal veins, and hypercoagulable state.

Fact: Diarrhea can cause a metabolic acidosis with an increased chloride level.

Fact: Pre-renal azotemia and acute glomerulonephritis can both have a low FENA. Acute glomerulonephritis will have an active urine sediment.

Fact: To delay onset of ESRD in patients with diabetic nephropathy: -Decrease BP to below 130/85 (will decrease proteinuria, prevent progression from microalbuminemia to overt nephropathy); Use ACE inhibitors; Dietary protein restriction to 0.6-0.8 g/k.

www.ingramcontent.com/pod-product-compliance
Lightning Source LLC
Chambersburg PA
CBHW071005180526
45168CB00003B/1302